RENAL DIET COOKBOOK FOR WOMEN

Women's Edition with Easy-to-Follow Recipes

FHARIE BELLY

Disclaimer:

The information provided in this book is for general informational purposes only. While every effort has been made to ensure the accuracy and completeness of the content, the author makes no representations or warranties of any kind, express or implied, about the completeness, accuracy, reliability, suitability, or availability of the information, products, services, or related graphics contained within this book.

Table of Contents

INTRODUCTION 1

A Tale of a Journey of Flavor 1

CHAPTER ONE 3

Understanding Renal Health for Women 3

1. Anatomy and Function of the Kidneys: 3

2. Common Renal Health Issues in Women: 3

3. Risk Factors for Renal Health Issues in Women: 4

4. Preventive Measures: 4

5. Regular Health Check-ups: 5

6. Seek Prompt Medical Attention: 5

CHAPTER TWO 6

Rise and Shine Breakfasts for Women 6

1. Overnight Oats with Chia Seeds and Berries 6

2. Vegetable Frittata 7

4. Sweet Potato Hash Browns 10

5. Spinach and Mushroom Omelets 11

6. Banana Walnut Pancakes (Low Potassium Version) 13

7. Egg Muffins with Spinach and Tomato 15

8. Cottage Cheese and Fruit Bowl......................... 16

CHAPTER THREE 18

Nourishing Lunches for Women's Wellness 18

1. Tuna Salad Lettuce Wraps 18

2. Mediterranean Quinoa Salad 19

3. Chicken and Vegetable Stir-Fry 20

4. Cauliflower Crust Pizza with Vegetables 22

5. Shrimp and Avocado Salad..................................23

6. Turkey and Cranberry Wrap 24

7. Grilled Vegetable and Hummus Sandwich 26

8. Spinach and Strawberry Salad with Balsamic Dressing..27

CHAPTER FOUR...29

Dinner Delights for Women's Health....................29

1. Lemon Garlic Roasted Chicken Thighs 29

2. Baked Cod with Tomato and Basil 30

3. Beef and Vegetable Kebabs 32

4. Eggplant Parmesan (Low Sodium Version) 33

5. Thai Peanut Tofu Stir-Fry.................................35

6. Stuffed Bell Peppers with Quinoa and Black Beans 37

7. Salmon Glazed in Teriyaki Sauce with Sesame-Coated Broccoli..39

8. Vegetable Stew with Herbed Couscous 41

CHAPTER FIVE 43

Snack Solutions for Women on the Go 43

1. Crunchy Cucumber and Hummus Slices 43

2. Edamame Sprinkled with Sea Salt................... 44

3. Fresh Guacamole Paired with Veggie Sticks.....45

4. Creamy Cottage Cheese with Pineapple Chunks 46

5. Rosemary Roasted Chickpeas............................47

6. Greek Yogurt Dip with Crudités 48

7. Almond Butter and Apple Slices 50

8. Rice Cake with Avocado and Tomato 51

CHAPTER SIX 53

Tempting Treats for Women's Wellness (Desserts) . 53

1. Berry Sorbet 53

2. Chocolate Avocado Mousse 54

3. Baked Apples with Cinnamon 55

4. Coconut Chia Pudding 56

5. Frozen Yogurt Bark with Fruit 58

6. Poached Pears in Red Wine 59

7. Mango Coconut Rice Pudding 61

8. Banana Bread (Low Potassium Version) 62

CHAPTER SEVEN 65

Balancing Social Life and Renal Health 65

1. Choosing Renal-Friendly Options at Restaurants:
.... 65

2. Navigating Buffets and Potlucks: 66

3. Strategies for Parties and Gatherings: 67

4. Tips for Traveling with Renal Diet Needs: 68

6. Creating a Supportive Social Network: 69

7. Incorporating Renal Diet into Family Meals: ...70

8. Celebrating Special Occasions Healthily: 71

CONCLUTION 73

2-Week Meal Plan 75

INTRODUCTION

"My Sister's Passion for Renal Diet Cookbook"

In the warmth of our home, bounded by the comforting aromas wafting from the kitchen, there resides a culinary virtuoso whose canvas isn't just a plate, but also the delicate balance of health and taste.

Meet my sister, Clara, a vibrant soul with an unwavering dedication to crafting delectable delights patched to the unique needs of women on a renal diet journey.

Clara's journey began not in a professional kitchen, but beside our grandmother's side, where she learned the transformative power of food. From those cherished moments, a passion for cooking bloomed within her, intertwining with her desire to make a difference in the lives of others.

It was when our aunt was diagnosed with kidney issues that Clara's path took a new turn. Witnessing the challenges our aunt faced in finding flavorful yet kidney-friendly recipes, Clara engaged in a mission to create a solution. Armed with her culinary skills and unwavering determination, she set out to develop a Renal Diet Cookbook lead specifically for women.

As Clara went deeper into her project, she embraced every aspect of it with fervor. She engage in understanding the intricacies of renal health, pouring over research papers and consulting with nutritionists to ensure her recipes not only riveted taste buds but also nurtured the body.

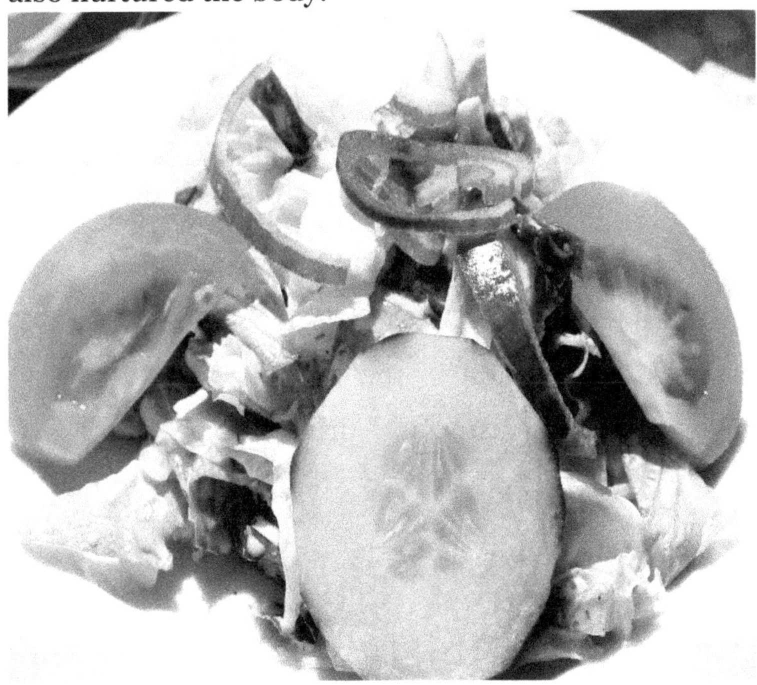

CHAPTER ONE

Understanding Renal Health for Women

These are some key points to consider:

1. Anatomy and Function of the Kidneys:

The kidneys are vital organs responsible for filtering waste products and excess fluids from the blood to form urine. They also help regulate electrolyte balance, blood pressure, and red blood cell production.

2. Common Renal Health Issues in Women:

• **Urinary Tract Infections (UTIs):** Women are more prone to UTIs due to their shorter urethra, which allows bacteria easier access to the bladder.

• **Kidney Stones:** Though both men and women can develop kidney stones, the risk factors may vary. Women with a history of urinary tract infections, obesity, or certain dietary habits may be more susceptible.

• **Chronic Kidney Disease (CKD):** CKD is a progressive loss of kidney function over time. Diabetes and high blood pressure are leading causes of CKD in women.

- **Autoimmune Diseases:** Conditions such as lupus and vasculitis can affect the kidneys, and these diseases are more common in women.

- **Pregnancy-related Kidney Issues:** Pregnancy can sometimes lead to complications such as gestational hypertension, preeclampsia, or eclampsia, which can affect renal health.

3. Risk Factors for Renal Health Issues in Women:

- **Hormonal Factors:** Hormonal changes during menstruation, pregnancy, and menopause can influence renal function and susceptibility to certain kidney conditions.

- **Pregnancy:** Women who have had multiple pregnancies or complications during pregnancy may have an increased risk of kidney issues later in life.

- **Age:** As women age, the risk of kidney problems, including CKD, tends to increase.

- **Family History:** A family history of kidney disease or related conditions can increase a woman's risk.

4. Preventive Measures:

- Stay Hydrated: Drinking plenty of water helps maintain kidney function and can help prevent kidney stones.

• **Healthy Diet:** Eating a balanced diet low in sodium and saturated fats and rich in fruits, vegetables, and whole grains can support overall kidney health.

• **Manage Chronic Conditions:** Keeping conditions like diabetes and high blood pressure under control through medication, lifestyle changes, and regular medical monitoring can help prevent kidney damage.

• **Regular Exercise:** Physical activity can help manage weight, blood pressure, and overall health, which in turn supports kidney function.

Avoiding Smoking and Excessive Alcohol: Smoking and heavy alcohol consumption can impair kidney function and should be avoided.

5. Regular Health Check-ups: Women should undergo regular health check-ups, including blood pressure monitoring and kidney function tests, especially if they have risk factors or a family history of kidney disease.

6. Seek Prompt Medical Attention: Any symptoms suggestive of kidney issues, such as changes in urination patterns, blood in the urine, persistent pain in the kidney area, swelling, or unexplained fatigue, should be promptly evaluated by a healthcare professional.

CHAPTER TWO

Rise and Shine Breakfasts for Women

1. Overnight Oats with Chia Seeds and Berries

Serving Size: 1 serving

Preparation Time: 5 minutes (plus overnight chilling)

Ingredients:

- 1/2 cup rolled oats
- 1 tablespoon chia seeds
- 1/2 cup unsweetened almond milk or low-fat milk
- 1/2 cup mixed berries (such as strawberries, blueberries, raspberries)
- 1 tablespoon honey or maple syrup (optional)
- Additional toppings: sliced almonds, shredded coconut, cinnamon (optional)

Instructions:

1. In a jar or container, combine rolled oats, chia seeds, almond milk, mixed berries, and honey or maple syrup (if using). Stir well to combine.

2. Cover the jar or container and refrigerate overnight, or for at least 4 hours, to allow the oats and chia seeds to soak and soften.

3. Before serving, stir the mixture. Add additional toppings if desired, such as sliced almonds, shredded coconut, or a sprinkle of cinnamon.

4. Enjoy cold as a nutritious and convenient breakfast option.

Nutritional Information (per serving):

Calories: 300, Protein: 9g, Carbohydrates: 50g

Fat: 7g, Fiber: 10g

2. Vegetable Frittata

Serving Size: 4 servings

Preparation Time: 30 minutes

Ingredients:

- 8 large eggs
- 1/4 cup milk or unsweetened almond milk
- 1 cup diced bell peppers (any color)
- 1 cup diced onions
- 1 cup diced tomatoes
- 1 cup chopped spinach or kale

- 1/2 cup shredded low-fat cheese (such as mozzarella or cheddar)
- Salt and pepper to taste
- Cooking spray or olive oil for greasing

Instructions:

1. Preheat oven to 350°F (175°C).

2. In a large bowl, whisk together eggs, milk, salt, and pepper until well combined.

3. Heat a skillet over medium heat and lightly grease with cooking spray or olive oil.

4. Add diced bell peppers and onions to the skillet and cook until softened about 3-4 minutes.

5. Add diced tomatoes and chopped spinach or kale to the skillet. Cook for another 2 minutes until vegetables are tender.

6. Pour the egg mixture over the cooked vegetables in the skillet. Sprinkle shredded cheese evenly on top.

7. Transfer the skillet to the preheated oven and bake for 15-20 minutes, or until the frittata is set in the center and the edges are lightly golden.

8. Remove from the oven and let it cool for a few minutes before slicing into wedges.

9. Serve hot as a satisfying and protein-rich breakfast option.

Nutritional Information (per serving):

Calories: 200, Protein: 15g, Carbohydrates: 8g

Fat: 11g, Fiber: 11g

3. Greek Yogurt Parfait with Almonds and Honey**

Serving Size: 1 serving

Preparation Time: 5 minutes

Ingredients:

- 1/2 cup Greek yogurt (unsweetened)
- 1/4 cup sliced almonds
- 1 tablespoon honey
- 1/4 cup mixed berries (such as strawberries, blueberries, raspberries)
- Optional: 1 tablespoon granola for added crunch

Instructions:

1. In a serving glass or bowl, layer Greek yogurt, sliced almonds, and mixed berries.

2. Drizzle honey over the top of the parfait.

3. Optionally, sprinkle granola over the layers for added texture.

4. Serve immediately as a protein-packed and delicious breakfast option.

Nutritional Information (per serving):

Calories: 300, Protein: 18g, Carbohydrates: 25g

Fat: 15g, Fiber: 4g

4. Sweet Potato Hash Browns

Serving Size: 2 servings

Preparation Time: 25 minutes

Ingredients:

- 2 medium sweet potatoes, peeled and grated
- 1/4 cup diced onion
- 1/4 cup diced bell peppers (any color)
- 1 tablespoon olive oil
- 1/2 teaspoon paprika
- 1/2 teaspoon garlic powder
- Salt and pepper to taste

Instructions:

1. Place grated sweet potatoes in a clean kitchen towel and squeeze out excess moisture.

2. In a large bowl, combine grated sweet potatoes, diced onion, diced bell peppers, paprika, garlic powder, salt, and pepper. Toss to coat evenly.

3. Heat olive oil in a skillet over medium heat. Add the sweet potato mixture to the skillet, spreading it out into an even layer.

4. Cook for 5-7 minutes on each side, or until hash browns are golden brown and crispy.

5. Remove from the skillet and drain on paper towels to remove excess oil.

6. Serve hot as a flavorful and nutritious breakfast side dish.

Nutritional Information (per serving):

Calories: 200, Protein: 3g, Carbohydrates: 30g

Fat: 8g, Fiber: 5g

5. Spinach and Mushroom Omelets

Serving Size: 1 serving

Preparation Time: 15 minutes

Ingredients:

- 2 large eggs
- 1/2 cup fresh spinach leaves, chopped
- 1/4 cup sliced mushrooms
- 1/4 cup diced onions
- 1 tablespoon olive oil
- Salt and pepper to taste
- Optional: shredded low-fat cheese

Instructions:

1. In a small bowl, whisk the eggs until well beaten. Season with salt and pepper.

2. Heat olive oil in a skillet over medium heat. Add diced onions and sliced mushrooms, and cook until softened about 3-4 minutes.

3. Add chopped spinach to the skillet and cook for another 1-2 minutes until wilted.

4. Pour the beaten eggs over the vegetables in the skillet, tilting the pan to spread them evenly.

5. Allow the eggs to cook undisturbed for a few minutes until the edges start to set.

6. Carefully lift the edges of the omelet with a spatula and tilt the skillet to let the uncooked eggs flow to the bottom.

7. Once the omelet is mostly set but still slightly runny on top, fold it in half with the spatula.

8. Cook for another 1-2 minutes until the eggs are fully cooked and the omelet is golden brown.

9. Optionally, sprinkle shredded low-fat cheese over the omelet before folding.

10. Slide the omelet onto a plate and serve it hot as a satisfying and protein-rich breakfast option.

Nutritional Information (per serving):

Calories: 200, Protein: 12g, Carbohydrates: 4g

Fat: 15g, Fiber: 2g

6. Banana Walnut Pancakes (Low Potassium Version)

Serving Size: 2 servings

Preparation Time: 20 minutes

Ingredients:

- 1 ripe banana, mashed
- 2 large eggs

- 1/2 cup almond flour
- 1/4 teaspoon baking powder
- 1/4 cup chopped walnuts
- Cooking spray or butter for greasing
- Sugar-free syrup or honey for serving (optional)

Instructions:

1. In a mixing bowl, combine mashed banana, eggs, almond flour, and baking powder. Mix until well combined.

2. Fold in chopped walnuts into the pancake batter.

3. Heat a skillet or griddle over medium heat and lightly grease with cooking spray or butter.

4. Pour about 1/4 cup of pancake batter onto the skillet for each pancake.

5. Cook until bubbles form on the surface of the pancake, then flip and cook until golden brown on both sides.

6. Repeat with the remaining batter.

7. Serve the pancakes hot, optionally drizzled with sugar-free syrup or honey.

Nutritional Information (per serving):

Calories: 350, Protein: 12g, Carbohydrates: 20g

Fat: 25g, Fiber: 5g

7. Egg Muffins with Spinach and Tomato

Serving Size: 6 muffins

Preparation Time: 25 minutes

Ingredients:

- 6 large eggs
- 1 cup fresh spinach, chopped
- 1/2 cup diced tomatoes
- 1/4 cup diced onions
- 1/4 cup shredded low-fat cheese
- Salt and pepper to taste
- Cooking spray or olive oil for greasing

Instructions:

1. Preheat oven to 350°F (175°C). Grease a muffin tin with cooking spray or olive oil.

2. In a mixing bowl, whisk the eggs until well beaten. Season with salt and pepper.

3. Divide chopped spinach, diced tomatoes, diced onions, and shredded cheese evenly among the muffin cups.

4. Pour the beaten eggs over the vegetable and cheese mixture in each muffin cup, filling them about 3/4 full.

5. Gently stir the mixture in each muffin cup with a toothpick to distribute the ingredients evenly.

6. Bake in the preheated oven for 15-20 minutes, or until the egg muffins are set and lightly golden on top.

7. Remove from the oven and let the muffins cool in the tin for a few minutes before carefully removing them.

8. Serve warm or at room temperature as a convenient and protein-packed breakfast option.

Nutritional Information (per muffin):

Calories: 9g, Protein: 7g, Carbohydrates: 2g

Fat: 6g, Fiber: 1g

8. Cottage Cheese and Fruit Bowl

Serving Size: 1 serving

Preparation Time: 5 minutes

Ingredients:

- 1/2 cup low-fat cottage cheese
- 1/2 cup mixed fresh fruit (such as berries, sliced banana, diced apple)

- 1 tablespoon chopped nuts (such as almonds, walnuts, or pecans)
- 1 teaspoon honey or maple syrup (optional)

Instructions:

1. in a bowl, spoon low-fat cottage cheese.

2. Top with mixed fresh fruit and chopped nuts.

3. Drizzle with honey or maple syrup if desired for added sweetness.

4. Serve immediately as a protein-rich and satisfying breakfast option.

Nutritional Information (per serving):

Calories: 220, Protein: 15g, Carbohydrates: 20g

Fat: 9g, Fiber: 3g

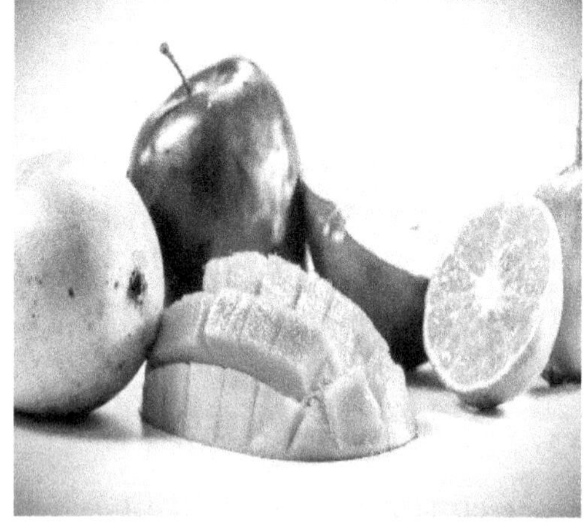

CHAPTER THREE

Nourishing Lunches for Women's Wellness

1. Tuna Salad Lettuce Wraps

Serves: 2

Prep Time: 15 minutes

Ingredients:

- 1 can (5 ounces) tuna, drained
- 2 tablespoons Greek yogurt
- 1 tablespoon lemon juice
- 1/4 cup diced celery
- 1/4 cup diced red onion
- Salt and pepper to taste
- 4 large lettuce leaves (such as romaine or butter lettuce)
- Optional toppings: sliced avocado, cherry tomatoes, shredded carrots

Instructions:

1. Combine drained tuna, Greek yogurt, lemon juice, diced celery, and diced red onion in a bowl.

2. Season with salt and pepper.

3. Spoon tuna mixture onto lettuce leaves.

4. Add optional toppings like avocado, cherry tomatoes, or shredded carrots.

5. Roll lettuce leaves into wraps.

6. Serve immediately for a light, protein-rich lunch.

Nutritional Info (per serving):

Calories: 150, Protein: 20g, Carbs: 4g

Fat: 5g, Fiber: 2g

2. Mediterranean Quinoa Salad

Serves: 4

Prep Time: 20 minutes

Ingredients:

- 1 cup cooked and cooled quinoa
- 1 cup cherry tomatoes, halved
- 1/2 English cucumber, diced

- 1/4 cup sliced Kalamata olives
- 1/4 cup crumbled feta cheese
- 2 tablespoons chopped fresh parsley
- 2 tablespoons extra virgin olive oil
- 1 tablespoon lemon juice
- Salt and pepper to taste

Instructions:

1. in a large bowl, mix quinoa, cherry tomatoes, cucumber, olives, feta cheese, and parsley.

2. Drizzle olive oil and lemon juice over the salad.

3. Season with salt and pepper.

4. Toss gently to combine.

5. Serve chilled or at room temperature.

Nutritional Info (per serving):

Calories: 220, Protein: 7g, Carbs: 25g

Fat: 11g, Fiber: 4g

3. Chicken and Vegetable Stir-Fry

Serves: 2

Prep Time: 25 minutes

Ingredients:

- 2 boneless, skinless chicken breasts, thinly sliced
- 2 cups mixed vegetables (bell peppers, broccoli, carrots, snap peas)
- 2 cloves garlic, minced
- 2 tablespoons low-sodium soy sauce
- 1 tablespoon hoisin sauce
- 1 tablespoon sesame oil
- 1 teaspoon cornstarch (optional, for thickening)
- Cooked brown rice or quinoa for serving

Instructions:

1. Mix soy sauce, hoisin sauce, sesame oil, and cornstarch in a bowl.

2. Cook chicken until browned and cooked through; set aside.

3. Stir-fry garlic and mixed vegetables until tender-crisp.

4. Return chicken to skillet; pour sauce over chicken and vegetables.

5. Cook until sauce thickens.

6. Serve over cooked brown rice or quinoa.

Nutritional Info (per serving, excluding rice/quinoa):

Calories: 250, Protein: 30g, Carbs: 10g

Fat: 9g, Fiber: 3g

4. Cauliflower Crust Pizza with Vegetables

Serves: 2

Prep Time: 40 minutes

Ingredients:

- 1 small head cauliflower, grated
- 1 egg
- 1/4 cup shredded mozzarella cheese
- 1/4 teaspoon dried oregano
- 1/4 teaspoon garlic powder
- Salt and pepper to taste
- 1/2 cup tomato sauce
- 1 cup mixed vegetables (bell peppers, mushrooms, onions)
- 1/4 cup shredded low-fat cheese (mozzarella or cheddar)

Instructions:

1. Prcheat oven to 400°F (200°C).

2. Microwave cauliflower for 5 minutes; let cool.

3. Mix cauliflower, egg, mozzarella cheese, oregano, garlic powder, salt, and pepper; form into crust.

4. Bake crust until golden brown.

5. Spread tomato sauce over the crust; top with mixed vegetables and low-fat cheese.

6. Bake until cheese melts.

7. Serve as a low-carb lunch option.

Nutritional Info (per serving):

Calories: 200, Protein: 10g, Carbs: 20g

Fat: 9g, Fiber: 6g

5. Shrimp and Avocado Salad

Serves: 2

Prep Time: 15 minutes

Ingredients:

- 8 ounces cooked shrimp, peeled and deveined
- 1 avocado, diced
- 1 cup mixed salad greens
- 1/4 cup cherry tomatoes, halved
- 1/4 cup cucumber, diced

- 2 tablespoons red onion, thinly sliced
- 2 tablespoons fresh cilantro, chopped
- 1 tablespoon olive oil
- 1 tablespoon lemon juice
- Salt and pepper to taste

Instructions:

1. In a large bowl, combine shrimp, avocado, mixed greens, cherry tomatoes, cucumber, red onion, and cilantro.

2. Drizzle olive oil and lemon juice over the salad.

3. Season with salt and pepper.

4. Toss gently to combine all ingredients.

5. Serve immediately as a refreshing and protein-packed salad.

Nutritional Info (per serving):

Calories: 250, Protein: 20g, Carbs: 10g

Fat: 15g, Fiber: 6g

6. Turkey and Cranberry Wrap

Serves: 1

Prep Time: 10 minutes

Ingredients:

- 1 large whole wheat tortilla
- 3 ounces sliced turkey breast
- 2 tablespoons cranberry sauce
- 1/4 cup mixed salad greens
- 2 tablespoons sliced almonds
- 1 tablespoon Greek yogurt (optional)
- Salt and pepper to taste

Instructions:

1. Lay the whole wheat tortilla flat on a clean surface.

2. Layer sliced turkey breast, cranberry sauce, mixed salad greens, and sliced almonds on the tortilla.

3. Optional: Spread Greek yogurt over the filling.

4. Season with salt and pepper to taste.

5. Roll up the tortilla tightly to form a wrap.

6. Slice in half if desired and serve immediately, or wrap in foil for later.

Nutritional Info (per serving):

Calories: 350, Protein: 25g, Carbs: 30g

Fat: 15g, Fiber: 5g

7. Grilled Vegetable and Hummus Sandwich

Serves: 2

Prep Time: 20 minutes

Ingredients:

- 1 zucchini, sliced lengthwise
- 1 yellow squash, sliced lengthwise
- 1 red bell pepper, seeded and quartered
- 1 small eggplant, sliced into rounds
- 4 slices whole grain bread
- 1/2 cup hummus
- 2 tablespoons balsamic vinegar
- 2 tablespoons olive oil
- Salt and pepper to taste

Instructions:

1. Preheat the grill or grill pan over medium-high heat.

2. Brush zucchini, yellow squash, red bell pepper, and eggplant slices with olive oil and season with salt and pepper.

3. Grill vegetables until tender and lightly charred, about 3-4 minutes per side.

4. In the meantime, toast whole-grain bread slices until golden brown.

5. Spread hummus evenly on each slice of toasted bread.

6. Arrange grilled vegetables on top of hummus.

7. Drizzle balsamic vinegar over the vegetables.

8. Top with remaining bread slices to form sandwiches.

9. Slice sandwiches in half if desired and serve immediately.

Nutritional Info (per serving):

Calories: 350, Protein: 10g, Carbs: 45g

Fat: 15g, Fiber: 10g

8. Spinach and Strawberry Salad with Balsamic Dressing

Serves: 2

Prep Time: 10 minutes

Ingredients:

- 4 cups fresh spinach leaves
- 1 cup sliced strawberries
- 1/4 cup sliced almonds
- 2 tablespoons crumbled feta cheese

- 2 tablespoons balsamic vinegar

- 1 tablespoon olive oil

- 1 teaspoon honey

- Salt and pepper to taste

Instructions:

1. In a large bowl, combine fresh spinach leaves, sliced strawberries, sliced almonds, and crumbled feta cheese.

2. In a small bowl, whisk together balsamic vinegar, olive oil, honey, salt, and pepper to make the dressing.

3. Drizzle the dressing over the salad and toss gently to coat evenly.

4. Serve immediately as a refreshing and nutritious salad.

Nutritional Info (per serving):

Calories: 200, Protein: 5g, Carbs: 15g

Fat: 10g, Fiber: 5g

CHAPTER FOUR

Dinner Delights for Women's Health

1. Lemon Garlic Roasted Chicken Thighs

Servings: 4

Prep Time: 10 minutes

Cook Time: 35 minutes

Ingredients:

- 4 chicken thighs, bone-in, skin-on
- 2 tablespoons olive oil
- 4 cloves garlic, minced
- Zest of 1 lemon
- Juice of 1 lemon
- 1 teaspoon dried oregano
- Salt and pepper to taste
- Fresh parsley, chopped (for garnish)

Instructions:

1. Preheat the oven to 400°F (200°C). Line a baking sheet with parchment paper.

2. In a small bowl, mix together olive oil, minced garlic, lemon zest, lemon juice, dried oregano, salt, and pepper.

3. Place the chicken thighs on the prepared baking sheet. Brush the lemon garlic mixture over the chicken thighs, coating them evenly.

4. Roast in the preheated oven for 30-35 minutes or until the chicken is cooked through and the skin is golden brown.

5. Garnish with chopped fresh parsley before serving.

Nutritional Information (per serving):

Calories: 300, Protein: 25g, Carbohydrates: 2g

Fat: 21g, Fiber: 0g

2. Baked Cod with Tomato and Basil

Servings: 2

Prep Time: 10 minutes

Cook Time: 20 minutes

Ingredients:

- 4 cod fillets
- 2 cups cherry tomatoes, halved

- 4 cloves garlic, minced

- 1/4 cup fresh basil leaves, chopped

- 2 tablespoons olive oil

- Salt and pepper to taste

- Lemon wedges (for serving)

Instructions:

1. Preheat the oven to 375°F (190°C). Lightly grease a baking dish with olive oil.

2. Place the cod fillets in the prepared baking dish. Season with salt and pepper.

3. In a bowl, mix together cherry tomatoes, minced garlic, chopped basil, and olive oil. Season with salt and pepper.

4. Spoon the tomato mixture over the cod fillets.

5. Bake in the preheated oven for 15-20 minutes or until the fish flakes easily with a fork.

6. Serve hot with lemon wedges on the side.

Nutritional Information (per serving):

Calories: 200, Protein: 25g, Carbohydrates: 4g

Fat: 9g, Fiber: 1g

3. Beef and Vegetable Kebabs

Servings: 4

Prep Time: 20 minutes

Cook Time: 10 minutes

Ingredients:

- 1 pound beef sirloin, cut into 1-inch cubes
- 1 red bell pepper, cut into chunks
- 1 green bell pepper, cut into chunks
- 1 red onion, cut into chunks
- 8 cherry tomatoes
- 8 button mushrooms
- 2 tablespoons olive oil
- 2 cloves garlic, minced
- 1 teaspoon dried thyme
- Salt and pepper to taste
- Wooden or metal skewers

Instructions:

1. If using wooden skewers, soak them in water for at least 30 minutes to prevent burning.

2. In a bowl, combine olive oil, minced garlic, dried thyme, salt, and pepper.

3. Thread beef cubes, bell peppers, onion chunks, cherry tomatoes, and mushrooms onto skewers, alternating the ingredients.

4. Brush the kebabs with the olive oil mixture, coating them evenly.

5. Preheat the grill to medium-high heat. Grill the kebabs for 8-10 minutes, turning occasionally, until the beef is cooked to your desired doneness and the vegetables are tender.

6. Serve hot as a delicious and nutritious dinner option.

Nutritional Information (per serving):

Calories: 300, Protein: 25g, Carbohydrates: 10g

Fat: 15g, Fiber: 3g

4. Eggplant Parmesan (Low Sodium Version)

Servings: 4

Prep Time: 20 minutes

Cook Time: 40 minutes

Ingredients:

- 1 large eggplant, sliced into rounds
- 1 cup marinara sauce (low sodium)

- 1 cup shredded mozzarella cheese (part-skim)

- 1/4 cup grated Parmesan cheese

- 1/4 cup breadcrumbs (whole wheat, optional)

- 1 tablespoon olive oil

- 2 cloves garlic, minced

- 1 teaspoon dried basil

- Salt and pepper to taste

- Fresh basil leaves (for garnish)

Instructions:

1. Preheat the oven to 375°F (190°C). Lightly grease a baking dish with olive oil.

2. Place eggplant slices on a baking sheet. Sprinkle with salt and let sit for 15 minutes to draw out moisture. Pat dry with paper towels.

3. In a small bowl, mix breadcrumbs (if using), minced garlic, dried basil, salt, and pepper.

4. Layer eggplant slices in the prepared baking dish. Top each slice with marinara sauce, shredded mozzarella cheese, Parmesan cheese, and breadcrumb mixture.

5. Repeat the layers until all ingredients are used, ending with a layer of cheese and breadcrumbs on top.

6. Bake in the preheated oven for 35-40 minutes or until the cheese is melted and bubbly and the eggplant is tender.

7. Garnish with fresh basil leaves before serving.

Nutritional Information (per serving):

Calories: 250, Protein: 10g, Carbohydrates: 20g

Fat: 15g, Fiber: 5g

5. Thai Peanut Tofu Stir-Fry

Serves: 4

Preparation Time: 15 minutes

Cooking Time: 15 minutes

Ingredients:

- 1 block (14 oz.) extra-firm tofu, pressed and cubed
- 2 tablespoons low-sodium soy sauce
- 2 tablespoons peanut butter
- 2 tablespoons lime juice
- 2 tablespoons honey or maple syrup
- 2 cloves garlic, minced
- 1 tablespoon grated ginger
- 2 tablespoons vegetable oil

- 1 red bell pepper, sliced

- 1 yellow bell pepper, sliced

- 1 cup broccoli florets

- 1 carrot, sliced

- Cooked brown rice or quinoa, for serving

- Optional garnish: crushed peanuts and chopped cilantro

Instructions:

1. Whisk together soy sauce, peanut butter, lime juice, honey (or maple syrup), garlic, and ginger in a small bowl for the sauce. Set aside.

2. Heat vegetable oil in a large skillet or wok over medium-high heat. Add tofu cubes and cook until golden brown on all sides. Remove tofu from the skillet and set aside.

3. In the same skillet, add sliced bell peppers, broccoli florets, and sliced carrots. Stir-fry for 5-6 minutes until vegetables are tender-crisp.

4. Return the cooked tofu to the skillet with the vegetables.

5. Pour prepared sauce over tofu and vegetables. Stir well to coat evenly.

6. Cook for another 2-3 minutes, or until the sauce is heated through.

7. Serve hot cooked brown rice or quinoa.

8. Optionally, garnish with crushed peanuts and chopped cilantro.

Nutritional Information (per serving, excluding rice/quinoa):

Calories: 300, Protein: 15g, Carbohydrates: 20g

Fat: 20g, Fiber: 5g

6. Stuffed Bell Peppers with Quinoa and Black Beans

Serves: 4

Preparation Time: 20 minutes

Cooking Time: 30 minutes

Ingredients:

- 4 bell peppers (any color), halved and seeds removed
- 1 cup cooked quinoa
- 1 cup black beans, drained and rinsed
- 1 cup corn kernels (fresh or frozen)
- 1/2 cup diced tomatoes
- 1/4 cup diced red onion

- 1/4 cup chopped fresh cilantro

- 1 teaspoon ground cumin

- 1/2 teaspoon chili powder

- Salt and pepper to taste

- 1/2 cup shredded cheddar cheese (optional)

Instructions:

1. Preheat the oven to 375°F (190°C) and lightly grease a baking dish.

2. In a large bowl, combine cooked quinoa, black beans, corn kernels, diced tomatoes, red onion, cilantro, ground cumin, chili powder, salt, and pepper.

3. Stuff each bell pepper half with the quinoa and black bean mixture.

4. Place stuffed bell peppers in the prepared baking dish.

5. Cover the dish with foil and bake in the preheated oven for 25 minutes.

6. Remove the foil, sprinkle shredded cheddar cheese over the stuffed peppers (if using), and bake for an additional 5 minutes or until the cheese is melted and bubbly.

7. Serve hot as a satisfying and nutritious dinner option.

Nutritional Information (per serving):

Calories: 250, Protein: 10g, Carbohydrates: 40g

Fat: 5g, Fiber: 10g

7. Salmon Glazed in Teriyaki Sauce with Sesame-Coated Broccoli

Serves: 4

Prep Time: 10 minutes

Cook Time: 15 minutes

Ingredients:

- 4 salmon fillets
- 1/4 cup low-sodium soy sauce
- 2 tablespoons honey or maple syrup
- 2 cloves garlic, minced
- 1 tablespoon grated ginger
- 1 tablespoon sesame oil
- 1 tablespoon rice vinegar
- 1 tablespoon cornstarch
- 1 tablespoon water
- 4 cups broccoli florets

- 1 tablespoon sesame seeds, for garnish

- Cooked brown rice for serving

Instructions:

1. Preheat the oven to 400°F (200°C) and line a baking sheet with parchment paper.

2. In a small saucepan, combine low-sodium soy sauce, honey (or maple syrup), minced garlic, grated ginger, sesame oil, and rice vinegar. Simmer over medium heat.

3. In a small bowl, create a slurry by mixing cornstarch with water. Stir the slurry into the simmering sauce until thickened, then remove from heat.

4. Arrange salmon fillets on the prepared baking sheet. Brush each fillet with the teriyaki sauce.

5. Surround the salmon with broccoli florets on the baking sheet. Drizzle a small amount of sesame oil over the broccoli and sprinkle sesame seeds on top.

6. Bake in the preheated oven for 12-15 minutes, or until the salmon is fully cooked and the broccoli is tender.

7. Serve hot alongside cooked brown rice.

Nutritional Information (per serving, excluding rice):

Calories: 300, Protein: 25g, Carbohydrates: 15g

Fat: 15g, Fiber: 5g

8. Vegetable Stew with Herbed Couscous

Serves: 4

Prep Time: 15 minutes

Cook Time: 30 minutes

Ingredients:

- 1 eggplant, diced
- 2 zucchinis, diced
- 1 yellow bell pepper, diced
- 1 red bell pepper, diced
- 1 onion, diced
- 2 cloves garlic, minced
- 2 cups diced tomatoes (canned or fresh)
- 2 tablespoons tomato paste
- 1 teaspoon dried thyme
- 1 teaspoon dried oregano
- Salt and pepper to taste
- 1 cup whole wheat couscous

- 1 1/4 cups vegetable broth

- 2 tablespoons chopped fresh parsley, for garnish

Instructions:

1. Heat olive oil in a large skillet over medium heat. Add diced eggplant, zucchini, bell peppers, onion, and minced garlic. Cook until vegetables begin to soften, approximately 5-7 minutes.

2. Stir in diced tomatoes, tomato paste, dried thyme, dried oregano, salt, and pepper. Simmer for an additional 10-15 minutes until vegetables are tender and flavors meld together.

3. In a separate saucepan, bring vegetable broth to a boil. Stir in couscous, cover, and remove from heat. Let stand for 5 minutes, then fluff with a fork.

4. Serve ratatouille over herbed couscous and garnish with chopped fresh parsley.

Nutritional Information (per serving):

Calories: 250, Protein: 7g, Carbohydrates: 50g

Fat: 2g, Fiber: 10g

CHAPTER FIVE

Snack Solutions for Women on the Go

1. Crunchy Cucumber and Hummus Slices

Time: 10 minutes prep

Serving Size: 2 servings

Ingredients:

- 1 large cucumber, sliced into rounds
- 1/2 cup hummus
- Optional toppings: paprika, sesame seeds, chopped parsley

Instructions:

1. Wash the cucumber thoroughly and slice it into rounds of even thickness.

2. Arrange the cucumber slices on a serving plate.

3. Spoon a dollop of hummus onto each cucumber slice.

4. Optionally, sprinkle paprika, sesame seeds, or chopped parsley over the hummus for added flavor and presentation.

5. Serve immediately as a refreshing and nutritious snack.

Nutritional Information (per serving):

Calories: 80, Protein: 3g, Carbohydrates: 9g

Fat: 4g, Fiber: 3g

2. Edamame Sprinkled with Sea Salt

Time: 5 minutes prep, 5 minutes cooking

Serving Size: 2 servings

Ingredients:

- 2 cups frozen edamame in the pod
- Sea salt to taste

Instructions:

1. Bring a pot of water to a boil over high heat.

2. Add the frozen edamame to the boiling water and cook for 5 minutes.

3. Drain the edamame and transfer them to a serving bowl.

4. Sprinkle sea salt over the edamame while they are still hot.

5. Toss the edamame gently to ensure even coating with sea salt.

6. Serve immediately as a nutritious and satisfying snack.

Nutritional Information (per serving):

Calories: 100, Protein: 8g, Carbohydrates: 8g

Fat: 3g, Fiber: 4g.

3. Fresh Guacamole Paired with Veggie Sticks

Time: 10 minutes prep

Serving Size: 2 servings

Ingredients:

- 2 ripe avocados
- 1 medium tomato, diced
- 1/4 cup finely chopped red onion
- 1 jalapeño pepper, seeded and finely chopped (optional)
- 2 tablespoons chopped fresh cilantro
- Juice of 1 lime
- Salt and pepper to taste
- Assorted vegetable sticks for dipping (carrots, celery, bell peppers, cucumber

Instructions:

1. Cut the avocados in half and remove the pits. Scoop the avocado flesh into a mixing bowl.

2. Mash the avocados with a fork until smooth or desired consistency.

3. Add diced tomato, chopped red onion, jalapeño pepper (if using), chopped cilantro, and lime juice to the mashed avocado.

4. Season with salt and pepper to taste.

5. Stir everything together until well combined.

6. Serve the guacamole immediately with assorted vegetable sticks for dipping.

Nutritional Information (per serving, guacamole only):

Calories: 160, Protein: 2g, Carbohydrates: 10g

Fat: 14g, Fiber: 7g

4. Creamy Cottage Cheese with Pineapple Chunks

Time: 5 minutes prep

Serving Size: 2 servings

Ingredients:

- 1 cup low-fat cottage cheese

- 1 cup fresh pineapple chunks

Instructions:

1. Divide the low-fat cottage cheese evenly between two serving bowls.

2. Top each bowl of cottage cheese with half of the fresh pineapple chunks.

3. Serve immediately as a creamy and refreshing snack.

Nutritional Information (per serving):

Calories: 140, Protein: 14g, Carbohydrates: 16g

Fat: 2g, Fiber: 2g

5. Rosemary Roasted Chickpeas

Time: 30 minutes

Serving Size: 4 servings

Ingredients:

- 1 can (15 ounces) chickpeas, drained and rinsed

- 1 tablespoon olive oil

- 1 teaspoon dried rosemary

- Salt and pepper to taste

Instructions:

1. Preheat the oven to 400°F (200°C).

2. Pat dry the chickpeas using a paper towel to remove excess moisture.

3. In a bowl, toss the chickpeas with olive oil, dried rosemary, salt, and pepper until evenly coated.

4. Spread the chickpeas in a single layer on a baking sheet lined with parchment paper.

5. Roast in the preheated oven for 25-30 minutes, shaking the pan halfway through, until the chickpeas are crispy and golden brown.

6. Remove from the oven and let cool slightly before serving.

7. Enjoy these crispy and flavorful roasted chickpeas as a nutritious snack!

Nutritional Information (per serving):

Calories: 150, Protein: 6g, Carbohydrates: 20g

Fat: 5g, Fiber: 6g

6. Greek Yogurt Dip with Crudités

Time: 10 minutes

Serving Size: 4 servings

Ingredients:

- 1 cup Greek yogurt
- 1 tablespoon lemon juice
- 1 clove garlic, minced
- 1 tablespoon chopped fresh dill
- Salt and pepper to taste
- Assorted crudités (carrots, cucumber, bell peppers, celery) for dipping

Instructions:

1. In a bowl, mix together Greek yogurt, lemon juice, minced garlic, chopped fresh dill, salt, and pepper until well combined.

2. Adjust seasoning according to taste preferences.

3. Serve the Greek yogurt dip with assorted crudités for dipping.

4. Enjoy this creamy and tangy dip with crunchy vegetables for a satisfying snack.

Nutritional Information (per serving):

Calories: 60, Protein: 6g, Carbohydrates: 4g

Fat: 2g, Fiber: 1g

7. Almond Butter and Apple Slices

Time: 5 minutes prep

Serving Size: 1 serving

Ingredients:

- 1 medium apple, sliced
- 2 tablespoons almond butter

Instructions:

1. Wash and core the apple, then slice it into thin wedges.

2. Spread almond butter on each apple slice.

3. Arrange the almond butter-topped apple slices on a plate.

4. Serve immediately as a wholesome and satisfying snack.

Nutritional Information (per serving):

Calories: 220, Protein: 5g, Carbohydrates: 25g

Fat: 12g, Fiber: 7g

8. Rice Cake with Avocado and Tomato

Time: 5 minutes prep

Serving Size: 1 serving

Ingredients:

- 1 rice cake
- 1/2 ripe avocado, sliced
- 1 small tomato, sliced
- Salt and pepper to taste
- Optional toppings: lemon juice, red pepper flakes, fresh herbs

Instructions:

1. Place the rice cake on a plate or flat surface.

2. Arrange the sliced avocado on top of the rice cake.

3. Place the tomato slices on top of the avocado.

4. Season with salt and pepper to taste.

5. Optionally, squeeze a little lemon juice over the toppings and sprinkle with red pepper flakes or fresh herbs for extra flavor.

6. Serve immediately as a light and satisfying snack.

Nutritional Information (per serving):

Calories: 130, Protein: 2g, Carbohydrates: 14g

Fat: 8g, Fiber: 4g

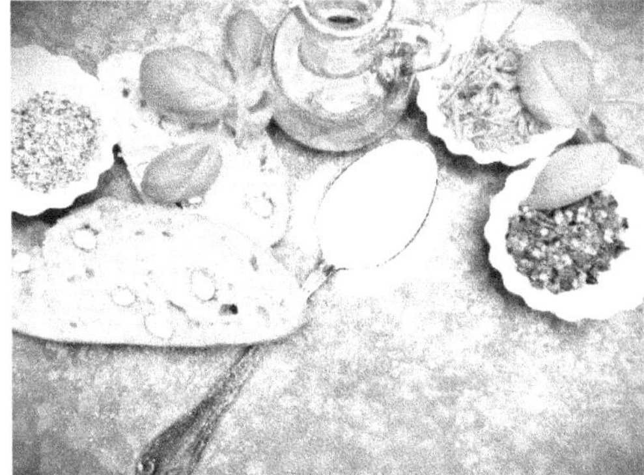

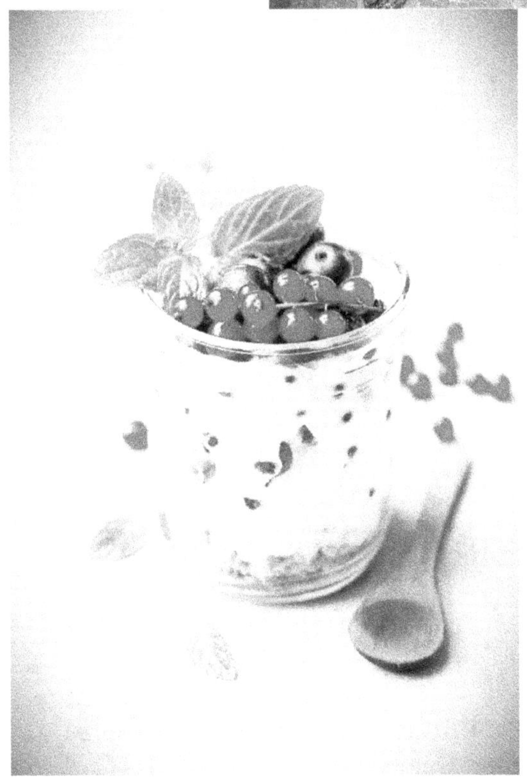

CHAPTER SIX

Tempting Treats for Women's Wellness (Desserts)

1. Berry Sorbet

Time: 5 minutes prep, 4 hours freezing

Serving Size: 4 servings

Ingredients:

- 2 cups mixed berries (such as strawberries, blueberries, raspberries)
- 1 tablespoon honey or maple syrup (optional)
- Juice of 1 lemon
- Fresh mint leaves for garnish (optional)

Instructions:

1. In a blender, combine the mixed berries, honey or maple syrup (if using), and lemon juice.

2. Blend until smooth.

3. Pour the mixture into a shallow dish and freeze for at least 4 hours or until firm.

4. Before serving, let the sorbet sit at room temperature for a few minutes to soften slightly.

5. Scoop into bowls, garnish with fresh mint leaves if desired, and serve immediately.

Nutritional Information (per serving):

Calories: 60, Protein: 1g, Carbohydrates: 15g

Fat: 0g, Fiber: 4g

2. Chocolate Avocado Mousse

Time: 10 minutes

Serving Size: 2 servings

Ingredients:

- 1 ripe avocado
- 2 tablespoons cocoa powder
- 2 tablespoons honey or maple syrup
- 1 teaspoon vanilla extract
- Pinch of salt
- Fresh berries for garnish (optional)

Instructions:

1. Scoop the flesh of the avocado into a blender or food processor.

2. Add cocoa powder, honey or maple syrup, vanilla extract, and a pinch of salt.

3. Blend until smooth and creamy.

4. Divide the mousse into serving bowls.

5. Garnish with fresh berries if desired.

6. Chill in the refrigerator for 30 minutes before serving.

Nutritional Information (per serving):

Calories: 200, Protein: 3g, Carbohydrates: 22g

Fat: 14g, Fiber: 7g

3. Baked Apples with Cinnamon

Time: 40 minutes

Serving Size: 2 servings

Ingredients:

- 2 apples (such as Granny Smith or Honeycrisp)
- 1 tablespoon honey or maple syrup
- 1 teaspoon ground cinnamon
- 1/4 cup chopped nuts (such as walnuts or almonds)
- Greek yogurt or whipped cream for serving (optional)

Instructions:

1. Preheat the oven to 375°F (190°C).

2. Core the apples and place them in a baking dish.

3. Drizzle honey or maple syrup over the apples.

4. Sprinkle cinnamon and chopped nuts over the apples.

5. Bake for 30-35 minutes or until the apples are tender.

6. Serve warm with a dollop of Greek yogurt or whipped cream if desired.

Nutritional Information (per serving):

Calories: 180, Protein: 3g, Carbohydrates: 32g

Fat: 7g, Fiber: 6g

4. Coconut Chia Pudding

Time: 5 minutes prep, 4 hours chilling

Serving Size: 2 servings

Ingredients:

- 1/4 cup chia seeds
- 1 cup coconut milk

- 1 tablespoon honey or maple syrup

- 1/2 teaspoon vanilla extract

- Fresh fruit for topping (such as berries or sliced banana)

- Shredded coconut for garnish (optional)

Instructions:

1. In a bowl, mix chia seeds, coconut milk, honey or maple syrup, and vanilla extract.

2. Stir well to combine.

3. Cover the bowl and refrigerate for at least 4 hours or overnight, until the mixture thickens and forms a pudding-like consistency.

4. Stir the pudding before serving to ensure an even texture.

5. Divide the pudding into serving cups or bowls.

6. Top with fresh fruit and shredded coconut if desired.

7. Enjoy this creamy and indulgent dessert!

Nutritional Information (per serving):

Calories: 250, Protein: 5g, Carbohydrates: 23g

Fat: 16g, Fiber: 10g

5. Frozen Yogurt Bark with Fruit

Time: 2 hours

Serving Size: 6 servings

Ingredients:

- 2 cups Greek yogurt
- 2 tablespoons honey or maple syrup
- 1 teaspoon vanilla extract
- Assorted fresh fruits (such as berries, sliced kiwi, and chopped mango)
- Optional toppings: shredded coconut, chopped nuts, dark chocolate chips

Instructions:

1. In a mixing bowl, combine Greek yogurt, honey or maple syrup, and vanilla extract. Stir until well mixed.

2. Line a baking sheet with parchment paper.

3. spread the Greek yogurt mixture evenly onto the parchment paper, about 1/4 inch thick.

4. Arrange the assorted fresh fruits on top of the yogurt mixture.

5. Sprinkle optional toppings like shredded coconut, chopped nuts, or dark chocolate chips over the fruits.

6. Place the baking sheet in the freezer for at least 2 hours, or until the yogurt bark is frozen solid.

7. Once frozen, break the bark into pieces.

8. Serve immediately as a refreshing and healthy dessert.

Nutritional Information (per serving):

Calories: 100, Protein: 8g, Carbohydrates: 15g

Fat: 1g, Fiber: 2g

6. Poached Pears in Red Wine

Time: 1 hour

Serving Size: 4 servings

Ingredients:

- 4 ripe pears, peeled and cored
- 2 cups red wine
- 1/2 cup honey or maple syrup
- 1 cinnamon stick
- 2 cloves
- 1 teaspoon vanilla extract
- Greek yogurt or vanilla ice cream for serving (optional)
- Fresh mint leaves for garnish (optional)

Instructions:

1. In a large saucepan, combine red wine, honey or maple syrup, cinnamon stick, cloves, and vanilla extract. Stir well.

2. Add the peeled and cored pears to the saucepan, making sure they are fully submerged in the liquid.

3. Bring the mixture to a gentle simmer over medium heat.

4. Reduce the heat to low, cover, and let the pears simmer for 30-40 minutes, or until they are tender when pierced with a fork.

5. Remove the pears from the poaching liquid and transfer them to serving plates.

6. Optionally, strain the poaching liquid to remove the spices and reduce it further on the stovetop to create a syrupy sauce.

7. Serve the poached pears warm or chilled, drizzled with the syrupy sauce, and accompanied by a dollop of Greek yogurt or a scoop of vanilla ice cream, if desired.

8. Garnish with fresh mint leaves for a pop of color.

Nutritional Information (per serving, without optional toppings):**

Calories: 200, Protein: 1g, Carbohydrates: 45g

Fat: 0g, Fiber: 5g

7. Mango Coconut Rice Pudding

Time: 40 minutes

Serving Size: 4 servings

Ingredients:

- 1/2 cup Arborio rice
- 2 cups coconut milk
- 1/4 cup honey or maple syrup
- 1 ripe mango, diced
- 1/4 cup shredded coconut
- 1 teaspoon vanilla extract
- Pinch of salt
- Ground cinnamon for garnish (optional)

Instructions:

1. In a saucepan, combine Arborio rice, coconut milk, honey or maple syrup, vanilla extract, and a pinch of salt.

2. Bring the mixture to a gentle simmer over medium heat, stirring occasionally.

3. Reduce the heat to low and let the rice cook for 30-35 minutes, or until it is creamy and tender, stirring occasionally.

4. Once the rice is cooked, remove the saucepan from the heat and stir in the diced mango and shredded coconut.

5. Let the rice pudding cool slightly before serving, allowing it to thicken further.

6. Divide the rice pudding into serving bowls and garnish with a sprinkle of ground cinnamon, if desired.

7. Serve warm or chilled, depending on preference.

Nutritional Information (per serving):

Calories: 300, Protein: 4g, Carbohydrates: 50g

Fat: 10g, Fiber: 3g

8. Banana Bread (Low Potassium Version)

Time: 1 hour 15 minutes

Serving Size: 8 servings

Ingredients:

- 2 ripe bananas, mashed

- 1/4 cup unsweetened applesauce

- 1/4 cup honey or maple syrup

- 1/4 cup almond milk

- 1 teaspoon vanilla extract

- 1 1/2 cups whole wheat flour

- 1 teaspoon baking powder

- 1/2 teaspoon baking soda

- 1/2 teaspoon ground cinnamon

- Pinch of salt

- Chopped walnuts or dark chocolate chips for topping (optional)

Instructions:

1. Preheat the oven to 350°F (175°C). Grease a loaf pan with cooking spray or line it with parchment paper.

2. In a mixing bowl, combine mashed bananas, unsweetened applesauce, honey or maple syrup, almond milk, and vanilla extract. Mix until well combined.

3. In a separate bowl, whisk together whole wheat flour, baking powder, baking soda, ground cinnamon, and a pinch of salt.

4. Gradually add the dry ingredients to the wet ingredients, stirring until just combined. Be careful not to overmix.

5. Pour the batter into the prepared loaf pan and spread it out evenly.

6. If desired, sprinkle chopped walnuts or dark chocolate chips over the top of the batter.

7. Bake in the preheated oven for 50-60 minutes, or until a toothpick inserted into the center comes out clean.

8. Remove the banana bread from the oven and let it cool in the pan for 10 minutes before transferring it to a wire rack to cool completely.

9. Once cooled, slice the banana bread and serve as a delicious and nutritious dessert or snack.

Nutritional Information (per serving):

Calories: 200, Protein: 4g, Carbohydrates: 40g

Fat: 3g, Fiber: 5g.

CHAPTER SEVEN

Balancing Social Life and Renal Health

Balancing social life with renal health requires careful consideration and planning, especially when it comes to dining out and attending social gatherings like buffets and potlucks. Here are some tips for women looking to maintain their renal health while enjoying social activities:

1. Choosing Renal-Friendly Options at Restaurants:

Research beforehand: Look up the menu online and identify renal-friendly options before going to the restaurant.

Opt for grilled or baked: Choose dishes that are grilled, baked, or roasted instead of fried, as these cooking methods usually involve less oil and are healthier for your kidneys.

Watch portion sizes: Restaurant portions are often larger than necessary. Consider sharing a dish with a friend or asking for a half portion to avoid overeating.

Be mindful of sauces and dressings: Many sauces and dressings are high in sodium and phosphorus, which can be harmful to renal health. Ask for sauces on the side and opt for low-sodium options when available.

Limit salt intake: Request dishes with no added salt or ask for dishes to be prepared with less salt. Avoid adding extra salt to the table.

2. Navigating Buffets and Potlucks:

Scan the spread: Before filling your plate, take a walk around the buffet table or potluck spread to see what options are available. This allows you to plan your meals and make healthier choices.

Choose wisely: Opt for renal-friendly foods such as fresh fruits and vegetables, lean proteins (like grilled chicken or fish), whole grains, and low-fat dairy products.

Control portion sizes: It can be tempting to sample everything at a buffet or potluck, but overeating can strain your kidneys. Use smaller plates and be mindful of portion sizes.

Be cautious of hidden ingredients: Some dishes may contain hidden ingredients that are high in sodium, potassium, or phosphorus. If you're unsure about a dish, ask the host or bring your renal-friendly dish to share.

Stay hydrated: Drink plenty of water to help flush out toxins and maintain kidney function, especially if you consume salty or high-protein foods at the event.

3. Strategies for Parties and Gatherings:

Communicate with the host: Inform the host of your dietary restrictions ahead of time so they can accommodate your needs or consider bringing a renal-friendly dish to share.

Eat before you go: Have a small, renal-friendly meal or snack before attending a party or gathering to help you resist the temptations of unhealthy foods.

Focus on socializing: Shift your focus from food to conversation and socializing. Engage in activities other than eating, such as dancing, playing games, or enjoying the company of friends and family.

BYOD (Bring Your Dish): If you're unsure about the food options available, bring your renal-friendly dish to ensure you have something safe to eat.

Limit alcohol and sugary drinks: Alcohol and sugary beverages can be dehydrating and may contain ingredients that are harmful to kidney health. Opt for water or other low-sugar, non-alcoholic options instead.

Plan ahead: Research restaurants and grocery stores at your destination that offer renal-friendly options. Consider packing snacks or meal replacements to have on hand in case suitable options are not readily available.

Pack smart: Bring a cooler or insulated bag to store perishable renal-friendly foods during travel. Pack renal-friendly snacks such as nuts, seeds, fresh fruits, and vegetables.

Stay hydrated: Traveling can be dehydrating, so be sure to drink plenty of water to support kidney function. Consider bringing a refillable water bottle and filling it up regularly.

Notify airlines or accommodations: If you have specific dietary needs, notify airlines or accommodations ahead of time so they can accommodate your requirements.

5. Making Modifications to Fast Food Chains:

Customize your order: Many fast-food chains offer customizable options. Ask for modifications such as removing cheese or sauce, opting for grilled instead of fried, or substituting sides for healthier options like salads or fruit cups.

Choose wisely: Look for menu items that are lower in sodium, phosphorus, and potassium. Grilled chicken sandwiches, salads with lean protein, and plain hamburgers without cheese or condiments can be better choices.

Read nutrition information: Check the nutritional information provided by fast-food chains to make informed choices about your meal. Look for options that are lower in sodium and other nutrients that may be harmful to kidney health.

Portion control: Fast-food portions are often larger than necessary. Consider splitting a meal with a friend or saving half for later to avoid overeating.

6. Creating a Supportive Social Network:

Educate your friends and family: Help those close to you understand your renal diet needs by providing them with information about your condition and dietary restrictions. This will enable them to support you better in social settings.

Join support groups: Seek out local or online support groups for individuals with kidney disease or those following renal diets. Connecting with others who share similar experiences can provide valuable support and advice.

Engage in kidney-friendly activities: Look for social activities that align with your renal diet needs, such as cooking classes focused on renal-friendly recipes, low-impact exercise groups, or support group meetings.

Communicate your needs: Don't be afraid to communicate your dietary needs and preferences when socializing with friends or attending gatherings. Most people will be understanding and accommodating if you explain your situation.

7. Incorporating Renal Diet into Family Meals:

Plan meals together: Involve your family in meal planning and preparation. Brainstorm renal-friendly meal ideas together and get everyone involved in cooking.

Focus on whole foods: Emphasize whole, unprocessed foods in family meals, such as fresh fruits and vegetables, lean proteins, whole grains, and healthy fats.

Offer variety: Keep meals interesting by experimenting with different flavors, spices, and cooking methods. Encourage family members to try new renal-friendly recipes and foods.

Provide education: Take the opportunity to educate your family about the importance of a renal diet and how it supports kidney health. Encourage open discussions about nutrition and wellness.

8. Celebrating Special Occasions Healthily:

Plan ahead: Anticipate special occasions and plan renal-friendly meals or snacks to enjoy during celebrations. Consider cooking at home or bringing a dish to share that aligns with your dietary needs.

Modify recipes: Adapt traditional recipes to make them more kidney-friendly by reducing sodium, phosphorus, and potassium content. Substitute ingredients as needed and focus on fresh, whole foods.

Practice portion control: Enjoy special occasion treats in moderation and be mindful of portion sizes.

Focus on savoring each bite and listening to your body's hunger and fullness cues.

Stay active: Incorporate physical activity into your celebrations by organizing outdoor games, going for a walk with friends or family, or dancing to your favorite music. Physical activity can help offset the effects of indulging in occasional treats.

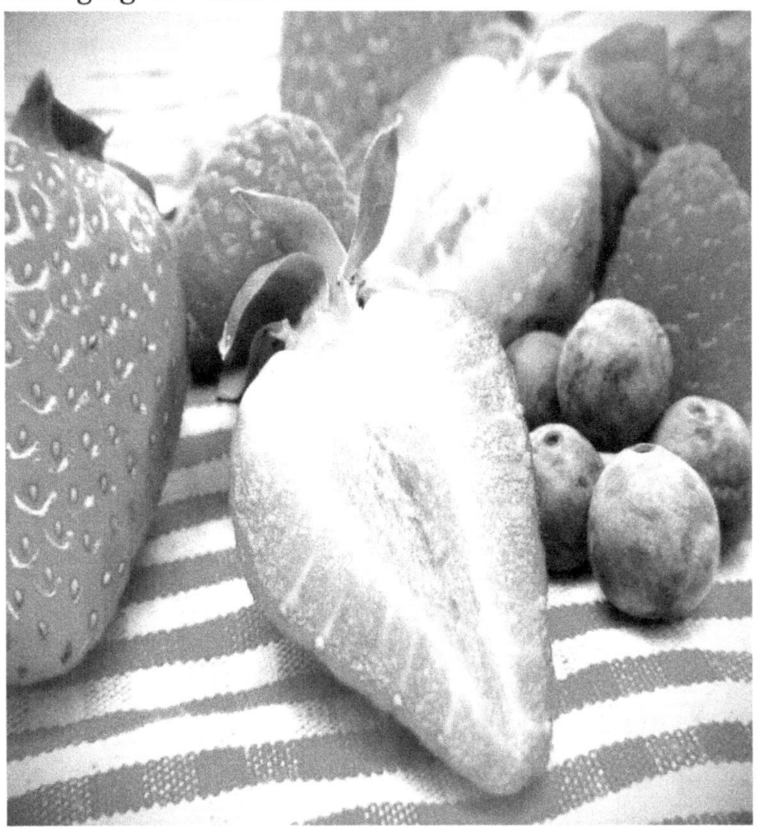

CONCLUTION

In the closing pages of "Renal Diet Cookbook for Women," I find myself reflecting on Clara's journey, a journey that began with a simple love for food and blossomed into a mission to empower women's health through flavorful, kidney-friendly cuisine.

As I turn the final pages of this culinary tale, I am reminded of the warmth of home, where the comforting aromas of Clara's creations fill the air, nurturing not only our bodies but also our spirits. Her dedication to crafting delectable delights patched to the unique needs of women on a renal diet journey is truly inspiring.

Through understanding the intricacies of renal health and embracing every aspect of her project with fervor, Clara has created more than just a cookbook – she has created a lifeline for women seeking flavorful yet nourishing meals. From Rise and Shine Breakfasts to Tempting Treats, each recipe is a testament to Clara's unwavering commitment to making a difference in the lives of others.

As I bid farewell to these pages filled with tempting recipes and valuable insights, let us carry Clara's passion and dedication with us on our journeys to health and wellness. May we continue to savor the flavors of life while nurturing our bodies with kindness and care, just as Clara has shown us through her culinary artistry.

In closing, let us remember that the journey of flavor is not just about what we eat, but also about the love and intention we infuse into every dish. Thank you, Clara, for sharing your passion with us and for reminding us that good food is indeed the ultimate nourishment for body and soul.

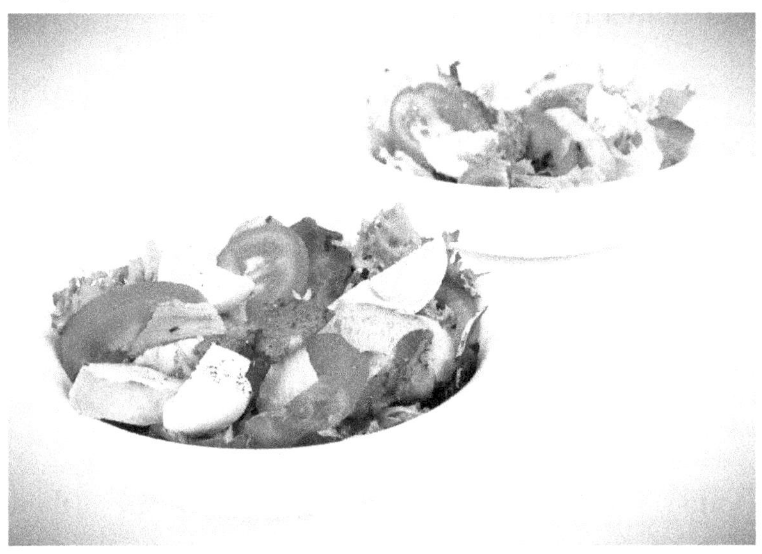

Week 1

Day 1: Monday

Breakfast: Overnight Oats with Chia Seeds and Berries

Lunch: Tuna Salad Lettuce Wraps

Dinner: Lemon Garlic Roasted Chicken Thighs with Quinoa and Steamed Green Beans

Day 2: Tuesday

Breakfast: Greek Yogurt Parfait with Almonds and Honey

Lunch: Mediterranean Quinoa Salad

Dinner: Baked Cod with Tomato and Basil served with Roasted Asparagus

Day 3: Wednesday

Breakfast: Spinach and Mushroom Omelets

Lunch: Chicken and Vegetable Stir-Fry with Brown Rice

Dinner: Beef and Vegetable Kebabs with Grilled Zucchini

Day 4: Thursday

Breakfast: Sweet Potato Hash Browns

Lunch: Cauliflower Crust Pizza with Vegetables

Dinner: Lentil and Vegetable Soup served with Whole Grain Bread

Day 5: Friday

Breakfast: Egg Muffins with Spinach and Tomato

Lunch: Turkey and Vegetable Lettuce Wraps

Dinner: Eggplant Parmesan (low sodium version) served with a side salad

Day 6: Saturday

Breakfast: Cottage Cheese and Fruit Bowl

Lunch: Spinach and Feta Stuffed Portobello Mushrooms

Dinner: Thai Peanut Tofu Stir-Fry with Brown Rice

Day 7: Sunday

Breakfast: Berry and Spinach Smoothie

Lunch: Avocado and Black Bean Salad

Dinner: Ratatouille with Herbed Couscous

Week 2

Day 8: Monday

Breakfast: Vegetable Frittata

Lunch: Tuna Salad Lettuce Wraps

Dinner: Lemon Garlic Roasted Chicken Thighs with Quinoa and Steamed Green Beans

Day 9: Tuesday

Breakfast: Greek Yogurt Parfait with Almonds and Honey

Lunch: Mediterranean Quinoa Salad

Dinner: Baked Cod with Tomato and Basil served with Roasted Asparagus

Day 10: Wednesday

Breakfast: Spinach and Mushroom Omelets

Lunch: Chicken and Vegetable Stir-Fry with Brown Rice

Dinner: Beef and Vegetable Kebabs with Grilled Zucchini

Day 11: Thursday

Breakfast: Sweet Potato Hash Browns

Lunch: Cauliflower Crust Pizza with Vegetables

Dinner: Lentil and Vegetable Soup served with Whole Grain Bread

Day 12: Friday

Breakfast: Egg Muffins with Spinach and Tomato

Lunch: Turkey and Vegetable Lettuce Wraps

Dinner: Eggplant Parmesan (low sodium version) served with a side salad

Day 13: Saturday

Breakfast: Cottage Cheese and Fruit Bowl

Lunch: Spinach and Feta Stuffed Portobello Mushrooms

Dinner: Thai Peanut Tofu Stir-Fry with Brown Rice

Day 14: Sunday

Breakfast: Berry and Spinach Smoothie

Lunch: Avocado and Black Bean Salad

Dinner: Ratatouille with Herbed Couscous.

9 798321 494752